No Ifs, Ands, or Butts

Find Linda on the Internet at:

Facebook: Linda T Gottlieb

Twitter: FITChicksRule

LinkedIn: Linda T Gottlieb

Blogging at: FITChicksRule.net/blog
www.FitTraining.net
www.FITChicksRule.net
www.MovingThroughCancer.com

All orders and inquiries for *No Ifs, Ands, or Butts* should be addressed to:

Linda T. Gottlieb
FIT Training LLC
www.FitTraining.net
(203) 877-5270

No Ifs, Ands, or Butts

How to Turn the Top 10 **EXERCISE** **EXCUSES** into Fitness Triumphs

LINDA T. GOTTLIEB, MA

Cover designed by Stacey Slimak.
Cover art designed by Randy Glasbergen.
Editorial assistance by Ronnie Ann Ryan.
Editing and page design by Katie Petito.

iUniverse, Inc.
Bloomington

No Ifs, Ands or Butts

How to Turn the Top 10 Exercise Excuses into Fitness Triumphs

You should not undertake any diet/exercise regimen recommended in this book before consulting your personal physician. Neither the author nor the publisher shall be responsible or liable for any loss or damage allegedly arising as a consequence of your use or application of any information or suggestions contained in this book.

iUniverse books may be ordered through booksellers or by contacting:

iUniverse
1663 Liberty Drive
Bloomington, IN 47403
www.iuniverse.com
1-800-Authors (1-800-288-4677)

Because of the dynamic nature of the Internet, any web addresses or links contained in this book may have changed since publication and may no longer be valid. The views expressed in this work are solely those of the author and do not necessarily reflect the views of the publisher, and the publisher hereby disclaims any responsibility for them.

ISBN: 978-1-4502-8582-7 (sc)
ISBN: 978-1-4502-8498-1 (ebk)

Library of Congress Control Number: 2011900433

Printed in the United States of America

iUniverse rev. date: 01/19/2011

For my amazing clients

You have demonstrated you have what it takes to significantly change your lives with strength and sparkle. What a brilliant display of personal power!

Cheers to you all!

Forward

By Melinda Irwin, PhD, MPH
Associate Professor of Epidemiology and Public Health
Yale School of Medicine

For over twenty years, I have conducted research on the benefits of exercise to promote health and prevent disease. My background in exercise physiology and cancer epidemiology has allowed me to examine first hand, the immediate (well, perhaps within three months) benefits of starting and maintaining an exercise program. Having conducted research for men and women with various diseases (diabetes, heart disease, breast and ovarian cancer), what I have noticed is that exercise not only improves the quality of life, but also the *quantity of life*!

Another important outcome is that study participants felt empowered by taking charge of their life. Their exercise routine allowed them to prioritize what is important to them and to live a fuller, happier life. But, most of them also experienced roadblocks or difficulties in the beginning and throughout their exercise journey. They all dug deep to find different strategies that helped them make it through the tough days and keep going.

This informative book by Linda Gottlieb focuses on a variety of simple strategies to help you stick with your exercise program; how to first recognize your excuses and then move past them. Her book is easy to follow, entertaining and works for both the beginner and advanced exerciser.

Linda has an extensive exercise background and experience coaching regular, every day people like you. She has led exercise trials and motivated men and women who have some of the most difficult barriers to overcome (e.g., surgery and treatment for cancer). Linda is an avid exerciser herself, yet acknowledges that she too has difficult days.

If you feel ready for a lifestyle change or need motivation and suggestions to get you back into your exercise program, then this book is for you!

Best wishes,
Melinda Irwin, PhD, MPH
Associate Professor
Yale School of Medicine

Contents

Introduction

I never set out to be a fitness professional. Loving movement, my early years were spent taking dance classes and losing myself in the beat of all kinds of music. In the early 1980s, I decided to become an aerobic dance instructor. If anyone had told me then that I would be in my 50s and still having fun with fitness, I would have laughed! However, through the decades I continued to learn about the awesome power of exercise, committed to living a fit life, and helped others do the same. The best part is watching people, maybe like you, be their *personal best*. That is my wish for you.

There you are sitting and reading a book about increased movement and personal energy! That's a funny contradiction, isn't it? But my friends and colleagues didn't think so, and their encouragement, along with decades of listening to my personal training clients, class participants, and workshop attendees, has resulted in this book.

As a student of behavior, I have always wondered what makes people do what they do. One day, becoming more fit will make it to the top of your to do list. That's great news! For most Americans, getting and staying fit requires only a slight change in daily actions: small, realistic steps that anyone can accomplish.

**"The best time to plant a tree is twenty years ago.
The second best time is now."
—Proverb**

This is your day! My intention is that you will use this book to challenge your exercise excuses and get started on your road to improved fitness and health. You'll find lots of ideas about how to begin from where you are today, without judgment. I promise to offer nurturing support, encouraging cheerleading, and the occasional tough love hug.

I have included research, assessments, and exercises to help you get to know yourself, along with some of my client's stories demonstrating how they have dramatically changed their lives by increasing physical activity. The aim of this book is to help you create your own roadmap to a fitter, healthier, and more joyful life. Maybe you'll even smile more along the way. If you move your body, there is no question that your life will improve. Read on and make it happen!

Let's Warm Up!

Traditionally, before starting exercise, you warm up. This chapter can be considered the "warm-up" for this book. Please read it first before skipping to any chapter of particular interest as it will help set the stage for what's to come.

"Exercise is like a four letter word! Why should I do any?"

First, let's start by dismissing the word entirely. That's right; you have permission to never even say the word "exercise" again. In this book, terms such as "physical activity" or "daily movement" are often exchanged for "exercise."

Take *Action* #1: Play the Name Game

Let's try to find some different words for "exercise." Don't forget to make them positive!

_____

_____

_____

_____

Great! Your first assignment is done! How easy was that? Simply by reframing a *word*, you can begin to leave the negative beliefs surrounding it behind and open your mind to a new way of thinking that just might lead to a more active, healthier you. Use your new words and see how they immediately change the way you view your relationship with this thing called "exercise."

! *You may not quite know it yet, but you are already on your way to the changes you want to make in your life. Hurray for you!*

Let's consider a strategy for simply moving more. The media, your doctor, and perhaps your family and friends remind you about the importance of _____ (insert one of your new, empowering words for "exercise"). The crisis of obesity and inactivity in this country is relatively new. It does not have to be your legacy unless you choose to make it so. Not only is daily physical activity good for your overall health, helping you to avoid or manage many serious diseases, it can increase your energy level and reduce stress.

"Those who think they have no time for exercise will eventually have to make time for illness."
—Edward Stanley

I like to say that your body is your own personal power plant. The time you put into daily activity will be returned in increased energy, health, focus, and joy that can be applied to things you *have* to do (work, caretaking, child raising) and things you *want* to do (playing with your children, social events, and hobbies). If you invest in the stock market you hope for a profitable return on investment, right? Be assured that even the most modest commitment to your health and fitness will offer a significant return on your investment. And what good is personal wealth without personal health?

! | *Life is a marathon, not a sprint.*

We'll be playing a few games throughout the book, starting with this one.

Take *Action* #2: Control Your Stress

We all have bad days, agreed? Here are two ways to react to a stressful day. Choose which option makes you feel empowered, strong, and in control:

1. Eating a handful of your favorite homemade cookies.
2. Walking a mile at a good pace.

I want to acknowledge right now that there is a place in life for cookies, ice cream, and potato chips. Just not the entire container and not every day. However, as your personal fitness motivator, I can almost guarantee that your logical mind selected option #2. Perhaps your emotional, experienced self laughed and said, "Sure #2 is a better answer, but I usually go down path #1." Don't worry! In sports parlance, life is a marathon, not a sprint, and you get to choose your pace and commitment level. You don't have to be perfect each and every day. Who is?

Also, keep in mind that moving more doesn't have to be a solitary activity. For some people (we will learn more about your exercise personality in a later chapter) taking a class, participating in a team sport, or walking with a buddy is a great way to keep the commitment going. Having a partner or group that is counting on you is a great way to share encouragement and stay motivated. When you decide to move more, you will become stronger and more flexible. You'll look great and feel even better. How empowered and confident do you feel when you look and feel great?

Are good health and fitness your #1 priority?

After more than 25 years as a fitness professional, I have heard perhaps every excuse for not exercising. I have also seen many of my friends, family, and coworkers age quickly, gain weight, become depressed and out of shape, and get sick due to lack of exercise. However (here's the tough love), there really are no valid excuses for not moving a little bit each day. Most people can accomplish some activity at any stage of life and benefit greatly from it.

So here's the hard question you must ask yourself: Do you really want to be fit and healthy? You might think this is a trick question, but it's not intended to be. Research proves time and time again that if something is a priority in your life it will simply get done.

Take *Action* #3: Prioritize Your Life

Jot down on the lines below your top three life priorities.

1. _____

2. _____

3. _____

Here's the reality: If you haven't put your personal health and fitness as a top priority, now is the time to decide how committed are you to this goal. Making the necessary changes to fit fitness into your life is critical to achieve good health. Whether your doctor tells you to lose weight and get more exercise or your family and friends think you ought to concentrate more on your health, it's you and only you that will make it happen. And you will only make it happen if it's a top priority.

! *Don't let black or white thinking get in your way.*

One of the most detrimental thought patterns, and the one that holds most people back, is called black-or-white thinking. Do any of these thoughts sound familiar?

"Either I lose 35 pounds for my sister's wedding or I'll die of embarrassment."

"If I don't lose this baby weight by the holidays, I'm not going to any parties!"

"I can't go to the alumni game unless I lose this last 20 pounds!"

The trouble is we *live* in the gray areas, where many unexpected things happen and little is black or white. Please accept that you live in the gray and that it's okay! I promise you, once you make daily fitness a "Fit It In" *game* rather than a line on what I call your "To Don't" list, your body will respond and your health will improve.

Everyone is busy. Declare that your health is a top priority, and I'll help you find ways to move more.

There are only two reasons why we do something: To avoid pain or experience pleasure

Think about increasing your daily activity in this way. Do you want to move away from pain—the physical distress of disease and illness, the emotional distress of depression and anxiety, and a life on the sidelines? Wouldn't you prefer the increased pleasure and happiness of healthy aging—a toned body and clothes that are stylish and fit you nicely?

You know what's really great? You are in charge, and you get to choose! Your subconscious mind will support your beliefs, no matter what they are. You get to select the movie that runs in your head, the biography you write about yourself, and the script your mind listens to daily.

! | *What you focus on unfolds.*

Why not edit the movie of your life to support a healthier, fitter you? The exciting news is that what you focus on is what unfolds for you. Focus on selecting healthier foods and finding fun ways to add more daily activity, and you will begin to manage your weight, increase your fitness level, and improve your outlook on life. Think like a fit, trim person and you can be one. What's better than that?

When I work with clients I lead them through an exercise about the power of a single thought. It goes like this:

> You have a thought.
> That thought creates a feeling.
> That feeling creates a behavior.
> That behavior creates a result.

Remember Stephen Covey's profound quote, "Begin with the end in mind"? Do you want to be a healthy, fit, happy person? Great! Let's start with that result and work back.

Take *Action* #4: Rewrite Your Mental Script

Jot down what behaviors a healthy, fit, happy person would have.

———————————————————————————

———————————————————————————

———————————————————————————

Great job! I did my homework, too. Here are a few behaviors I thought of for you: walk every day, get plenty of restful sleep, smile a lot, choose lots of fresh fruits and vegetables for meals, and think positive thoughts about body image.

Take a moment to write down what it might feel like if you consistently behaved like your list above.

———————————————————————————

———————————————————————————

———————————————————————————

———————————————————————————

You might feel strong, purposeful, in control, and hopeful. Do you like how that feels? Are you smiling?

Let's continue to work the model backward to the beginning, where all results come from. As this fit and healthy person, what thoughts might run through your head (creating a new script) that would trigger the behaviors listed above and deliver the results you seek?

_____

_____

_____

_____

Does your new script include:
- Loving yourself? Sure!
- Opening up to new and exciting possibilities in your life? Absolutely!
- Viewing the world with optimism about your future? Yes!

Do you usually have these kinds of feelings on a daily basis? No? Well, then why not start incorporating them today? Play this game often to see what kind of results you can manifest.

Are you having a bit of difficulty believing that thoughts create your behaviors, and ultimately, results? This next task will help.

Take *Action* #5: Think Yourself Thin

Find a time when you are alone and not distracted. Close your eyes, and take a deep breath. Think of a just-picked, farm-fresh lemon. Yes, the yellow pungent fruit that smells so fresh and clean. Picture the brilliant, sunny yellow, bumpy skin, the tart surprise of a fresh slice, and the zesty burst of flavor of tangy, icy lemonade.

Is your mouth watering? Got a pucker going? Eureka! It's a physiological reaction, but the lemon appeared only in your imagination. It was the *thought of the lemon* that created the physical reaction!

I bet you can think of many other thoughts that trigger results. It's the negative thoughts that usually derail the best intentions regarding fitness and weight management. That's why so much of my work is helping clients create new mental scripts so their desired results can be obtained. Our brains are intricate, powerful mechanisms. Why not use yours to get fitter and healthier and redefine how you think about yourself and fitness?

Sorry, you are NOT excused!

Last, let me just holler out with my best boot camp sergeant's voice "You are NOT excused!" Exercise excuses may shorten your life and make it less joyful.

Human beings don't like pain, but we do love pleasure. Excuses are used to wiggle out of doing something you don't want or like to do and provide a justification for it. It's my belief that the excuses you make up and tell yourself might be the most detrimental of all. Why? Because at some point, you start believing them!

Take *Action #6*: Word Reactions

Jot down all the things you think about each word below. Don't think too hard. I want your first impressions.

Gym _____

Workout _____

Exercise _____

Muscle _____

Fit _____

Did your list look anything like:

Gym: Fun!
Workout: Energy!
Exercise: Life!
Muscle: Strength!
Fit: Healthy!

Or more like:

Torture!
Boring!
Hurts!
Big!
Someone else!

Your candid responses are simply the unedited way you think of exercise, but you can decide to alter these assumptions. As you continue on, remember this . . . *to change your body you must change your mind.*

You've done a great job warming up for the exercise excuses in the remainder of this book. You now know what some of your beliefs are, that fitness is an important priority in your life, and that you can make the changes you want. Let's get going and turn your exercise excuses into fitness triumphs!

Exercise Excuse #10:

"I can't afford an expensive gym membership/equipment/gear."

"Prosperity begins with feeling good about myself. Therefore, I prosper in all areas of my life. I always have everything I need."
—Louise Hay

Many advertisers would like you to believe that the answer to your fitness prayers is to invest in their gadget, program, or membership.

The next time you are captivated by these promises, take a moment to look around your home for previously purchased fitness items that are simply collecting dust. It's a joke inside the fitness industry (but so true!) that most home treadmills are used as clothes hangers rather than for exercise.

Of course, a good fitness option is to join a gym, health club, or country club. The local community centers, hotels, and even your corporate fitness facility can be affordable options, along with some national chain fitness centers. Remember, the most glamorous facilities usually attract those that need them the least.

However, if the cost is still out of your budget, let's deal directly with what is really required as a start-up fitness investment.

- Walking is the #1 fitness activity in the world, and you can do it too. You can walk anytime, anywhere. All you need is a good pair of sneakers to begin your fitness program.
- Dumbbells can be used for a variety of exercises and are also inexpensive. They can be purchased at a discount retailer or neighborhood garage sale. Resistance bands (which you may already have from physical therapy) or even soup cans right out of your pantry can work too.
- Visit your local library and check out their videos on dance aerobics, cardio-kickboxing, yoga, or tai chi, which are all perfect for the home exerciser. The Internet, YouTube™ in particular, has some quick and simple videos to learn from. I recommend you first check the credits to make sure they are recorded by a certified fitness professional.

From the minute you wake up until the moment your head hits the pillow at night, there are opportunities for increased physical activity, with or without props. In the 1940s, inmates entered prison with deconditioned physiques and were released in great physical shape. They didn't have gyms back then or any equipment. They used their free time (they had quite a lot!) and their own muscles as resistance (called isometrics) to strengthen, tone, and build muscle. You can do it, too, and without the prison sentence.

At home, your next workout may be no farther away than your kitchen, laundry room, or basement stairs. You can easily add a few minutes of cardiovascular movement (cardio or aerobic exercise that raises your heart rate), strength training (exercise that makes your muscles work harder, get and stayed toned), and stretching for flexibility into your schedule every day.

You don't have to spend a penny to set up your own House Work-Out. Here are some sample exercises you can do:

1. **Start with a few minutes of cardio:** Walk briskly through your home, from room to room. Listening to energizing music helps the effort by keeping you on an upbeat stride. March, dance, jump to the beat. Need to take a phone call? Mute the music and pace. Don't forget to clean the house; it burns tons of calories. Chase the dust bunnies and burn the fat. You'll have more energy almost immediately.

2. **Use your stairs:** Think of them as a free Stairmaster™. Use them for intense interval training by taking one handful of laundry at a time up and down to the washer. The larger the family the better the workout! Push from the heel, not the knee, and alternate between going up every step and skipping a step. When you get stronger, don't hold on to the handrail. Keep your heart rate up, but stop if you feel dizzy. As you continue to improve, leave the laundry in the basket and walk up and down the stairs with soup cans.

3. **For strength, pretend to "sit" on a phantom chair:** To strengthen your thighs, press your back against a solid wall, with your knees bent over your feet at a 90-degree angle, your thighs taking your weight. (You'll look like you're sitting on a chair.) Hold until your thighs tell you to it's time to get up. (They will!) "Sit" longer each time.

4. **Use the kitchen counter for isometric push-ups:** For your chest and back, stand an arms-length away from a sturdy counter, desk, or table. Straighten your body and stand on your toes. Keeping your body rigid, bend your elbows to let your body lean toward the counter, heels lifting. Do not

let the shoulders hunch or the belly sag. Push yourself back up to standing by straightening the arms. You can also do push-ups against a solid wall.

5. **Abdominal exercises:** Do you have children, a spouse, or pet to pick up after? Sit on the floor with your back straight, with feet down and knees bent, and lean back just as far as comfortable, exhaling and holding in your belly. Turn, stretch, and reach for the first object/toy/sock, collect it, then sit up straight and inhale. Repeat until the floor is clean in your immediate reach, reposition yourself, and continue. Whew! After you get stronger, use those soup cans held close to your chest for increased resistance (or held away from your body to intensify even more) and feel how much more you get out of this exercise.

6. **Feeling strong and sassy?** Collect two plastic gallon milk containers, fill with water, and lift. They weigh approximately five pounds, more when filled with sand. Use for bicep curls and tricep drops (two hands holding one container lifting above and lowering behind your head). Without the weight, contract the muscles (like Popeye) and do it the isometric way.

7. **Cool-down stretch:** Use a bath towel folded the long way as a rope and hook it under one foot while lying on the floor. Try to straighten your leg and use the towel to assist while gently pulling your leg slowly (never bouncing) toward your face. Hold and breathe, then repeat on the other side.

8. **Hamstring stretch:** Use those same water-filled gallon jugs for a dead lift stretch by standing tall, keeping shoulders and chin relaxed and back. Holding one gallon

in each hand, keep arms straight down and bend slowly and gently from the waist. Allow the weight of the jugs to help you relax forward into a wonderful hamstring stretch. Hold at the point you are most comfortable and breathe. With your back straight and chin up, lift from the waist until you are again standing tall. Repeat several times. Contract your arm muscles (isometrics again) to replace holding a weight.

Get creative. What other places in or outside your home, or chores do you consider mundane that have fitness potential? Whether it's around the living room or around the block, it's free!

Corporate cube dwellers and road warriors

I didn't forget about office workers. Did you know that research has proven corporate casual dressing can help you increase the exercise you get in your day? This is great news!

Remember the 80s workplace? I do. Ladies wore high heels and suits with skirts, and men were all decked out in a button-down shirt and tie and those expensive leather dress shoes (not as comfy as sneakers)—maybe even a suit! Those of you who remember these days recall how difficult it was to simply move around the workspace, let alone climb stairs, go for a fast walk at lunch, or lift heavy catalogs, books, or other office paraphernalia.

However, in those days you were more likely to get out of your chair to walk to a coworker to have a conversation. The advent of e-mail and instant messaging in business environments has led to a 10-pound increase in weight and a significant decrease in health.

So ditch the high heels and take advantage of your dressed-down attire to ramp up your office fitness and move.

The American Council on Exercise, America's nonprofit fitness advocate, reported on a study comparing how wearing casual clothing vs. wearing conventional business attire affects daily physical activity levels. The study examined healthy men and women who wore a step counter two days a week (one day dressed in normal work attire and the other dressed in jeans) for two weeks.

Researchers found that workday physical activity levels increased when casual clothing was worn. Specifically, study participants took an average of 491 (or 8%) more steps on Jeans Day than on those days when they wore business attire. That is an average of 2.85 miles vs. 2.64 miles walked, burning an average of 25 additional calories. Doesn't sound like much? Keep reading.

Wearing casual clothing every day for 50 weeks translates into burning an additional 125 calories per week and 6,250 calories per year. Considering you must burn 3,500 calories to lose one pound, the added activity from casual workdays could potentially offset the average annual weight gain (i.e., 0.4 to 1.8 pounds) experienced by American adults!

This study was groundbreaking as it isolated a simple factor of a clothing choice and its impact on fitness levels. I bet you even know folks who work in cities and wear sneakers to walk from the train or other mass transportation who can vouch for the improvement in their fitness level.

Cedric Bryant, PhD, chief exercise physiologist at ACE says, "Over the last 25 years, advances in technology combined with our hectic lifestyles have helped to virtually eliminate physical activity from our daily routines." He goes on to advocate "Wearing casual, comfortable clothes to work may be an easy way to encourage us to put physical activity back into our daily lives."

It's a sign . . .

In another study, researchers at the University of Pennsylvania devised an experiment focused on using the stairs vs. the escalator in a public transportation center. The observers counted how many people opted for the escalator (a lot!) rather than the stairs.

Next the researchers posted a sign at the escalator telling people to take the stairs "for a healthy heart." Immediately after the sign was posted, many more people took the stairs, and continued to do so until the sign was removed. Stair usage doubled during this time compared to the baseline measurement. After the sign was removed, stair use declined rapidly until within a few months, the commuters were back to taking the escalator.

Sometimes all we need are simple reminders to change daily habits and improve our health! Taking the stairs makes good sense and is a free fitness option.

Successtimonial: You ride. I'll take the stairs.

Sara, an executive recruiter in Manhattan challenged my "take the stairs" suggestion one day. "I work on the 27th floor!" she said with a defiant look on her face, which clearly communicated that hiking 815 steps to her office was out of the question. Of course, it's my job to help folks move past limiting beliefs, so I suggested she begin conservatively, and take the elevator to the 26th floor and walk the one remaining flight. Sara's reply? "Huh! I never thought of that. Now, that I can do!"

Take *Action* #7: Small Steps Make a Big Difference

Try one or more of the following:

- Park (safely) one to three blocks away from your destination and walk.
- Visit the grocery store (or large retail store) and walk around the inside perimeter at least once before making your purchases.
- Locate fitness equipment in your home (or improvise with the household ideas provided earlier) to create a beginner strength program.

I like to say, "repetition is the mother of results," so keep at it!

Exercise Excuse #9:

"I get enough exercise in my day."

"If your dog is fat, you're not getting enough exercise."
—Unknown

Uh oh . . . let's bust this myth right now. Most American's *do not* get enough exercise in a normal day. Even busy moms realize when they measure their activity using an accelerometer (high-tech calorie counter), step counter, or simple time journal that they are not as active as they thought.

As a matter of fact, Americans commonly overestimate their daily activity and underestimate the amount of food and number of calories they consume. This is a dangerous equation that has left the country with a health crisis. Has it created a personal crisis for you too?

Conversely, some folks in professions such as lawn care, postal/package delivery, and construction do move a lot. Adding a strength program, stretching/flexibility activity, and cardiovascular exercise that raises the heart rate to the optimal zone can augment the activity these folks already do in their work day and round out a lifetime fitness plan. How does your day measure up?

Take *Action* #8: Are You Active?

Take five minutes to review your day yesterday. Use the personal time journal provided to jot down how you spent your day, on the scale of moving (answer yes or no). Remember that each day has 1,440 minutes and 360-480 minutes are spent sleeping.

Your Personal Time Journal

Date: _____   Day of Week: _____

Time	Activity	Moving?	Not moving?
8 a.m. – noon	Desk work/meetings		195 min.
7:53 – 8 a.m.	Walk from car to office	7 min.	

TOTAL TIME _____

What did you learn? How much time do you sit in front of your computer, sitting in meetings, making phone calls, or commuting? Don't forget the minutes (or is it hours?) you're glued to the TV, engrossed in a new book, or playing cards.

Here's a riddle:
Q: How do you waste an hour?
A: Checking your e-mail for five minutes.

You get the hang of it. Now, don't beat yourself up. Give yourself credit for *any* activity you engaged in during the day, even if you did not exercise in a structured way. Knowing where you stand as a baseline is the first important step in creating a more active you.

Remember, you get "Kudos!" for walking up the stairs (or a few flights before hopping on the elevator), "Excellent work!" for walking to a colleague's office instead of e-mailing them, or "Yeah for you!" if you took a walk to get lunch or water. All of that time belongs in the "moving" column.

Add up those minutes, along with the ones you spent on stationary activities. Hmm, are the numbers shocking? If so, keep reading!

The lesson is that you *can* rearrange some of your day for fitness, and do it without a gym membership, expensive equipment, or wearing uncomfortable clothes!

If you are already physically active during your day, terrific! You need only to make sure you get your heart rate up. Use the "Talk Test" to tell if you are working out at a proper intensity. Your workout should be intense enough to make you breathe deeply and feel a little winded, but you should still be able to carry on a conversation while you exercise. If you don't have enough breath to get the words out, you're working too hard, so slow down a bit. Back off until you can speak comfortably. On the other hand, if you don't feel winded at all, you can increase your intensity by going faster or walking uphill rather than on a flat surface.

If you are getting at least 20-30 minutes per day where your heart rate is elevated as described, you are probably getting enough cardiovascular exercise. If not, add some extra minutes of vigorous movement. Don't forget to lift some heavier weights (I say "No Barbie weights!"), and increase your stretch time.

Successtimonial: Tale of a mover and a shaker

John thought that his sales job kept him moving all the time, and he was sure the step counter he wore and time journal he completed would validate his assumptions. John quickly learned that although he is quite active on client appointment days (walking from a remote area of the parking lot, carrying marketing materials, and taking the stairs when possible), most of his week was spent driving, sitting at the computer, and talking on the phone. Seeing the real data (think of that old adage "what you measure you can change") allowed John to be open to recommendations for slight alterations in his day that added more movement.

Take *Action* #9: Reward Yourself

Before beginning this task, complete the personal time journal for an average weekday and weekend day (they can be quite different). Purchase a step counter (www.accusplit.com) to collect additional baseline data.

1. Find three times when you can alter your behavior to increase your activity, such as pacing while on the telephone, sitting on a fitness ball instead of a chair at your desk, taking a walk, or stretching for every 30-45 minutes of computer work.
2. Celebrate the small changes you make by buying a new CD, getting a massage, or taking a walk on the beach. No food rewards, please!

We know that moderate amounts of physical activity have been shown to improve health, yet more than 65% of Americans do not get enough and 25% are completely inactive. How do you compare?

Using a simple step counter can provide the information to validate your activity, encourage you, help track success, and get you on or back on track when best-laid plans go awry. My clients wear a step counter every day, not only to stay focused, but to see real progress.

How do your steps compare? The chart below gives you some idea of your current level of physical activity.

Fitness Level	Steps Per Day
Very inactive	2,500 or less
Inactive	2,501-5,000
Moderately active	5,001-7,500
Active	7,501-10,000
Very active	10,000 or more

Some step facts:
- Most Americans are in the very inactive category.
- 1 mile = 2,000-2,500 steps
- 4.5 miles = 10,000 steps
- One city block is about 200 steps
- Nine holes of golf with no cart = 8,000 steps
- Most people walk approximately 1,200 steps in 10 minutes (time it yourself for your baseline number).

Exercise Excuse #8:

"I'm healthy, so I don't need to exercise."

"Even if you are on the right track, you'll get run over if you just sit there."
—Will Rogers

Congratulations! If you are healthy, being fit and staying physically active will keep you there. Be proud of your attention to this critical life project called "My Health."

Spend some time creating your long-term health and wellness strategy. Most people take more time planning a tropical vacation than planning for the most important aspect of their life: a strong, healthy body and mind.

You wouldn't let your car run without any engine oil, let the fenders rust, or the tires go flat, would you? So why spend years assuming that you are entitled to good health and fitness if you do nothing to retain or maintain it? Also, wearing a size 2 dress or 34 pants is no guarantee of good health. It doesn't relate to having a strong heart, healthy blood pressure, or the strength to lift your grandchild without hurting your back.

The value of exercise in growing older

Dr. Paul Batman, sports scientist and director of the Fitness Institute of Australia says, "I think we convince ourselves that at 20, 30, or 40 we are still young and healthy, so we don't need to exercise." He goes on to remind us that "Everything we do in our youth comes back to haunt us in later years. It's not as if when we turn 40 everything deteriorates. It's 40 years of living that has contributed to the deterioration."

"After you turn 30, if you are inactive, you start to lose your type-two muscle fibers—the ones that give you strength and power. This means you are less able to ward off frailty in old age. You can maintain those muscle fibers that allow you to remain strong," Batman says.

Successtimonial: A not-so-pleasant surprise

Cheree was 42 when we met at a business function. She discounted her need for exercise since she felt young, healthy, and looked great in her clothes. However, after a routine medical exam, Cheree was shocked learn that she had osteopenia, a precursor to osteoporosis. She found out that thin people are at increased risk of osteoporosis and high blood pressure. Most times the symptoms of serious medical conditions are not obvious to the individual. For Cheree, the introduction of weight-bearing exercise (such as walking, running, and strength training) helped her begin to manage this health challenge. Cheree is 48 now, in the best shape of her life, and has stabilized her osteopenia.

Whatever your age or current health situation, exercise is an important part of a joyful life plan. Take a few moments to think about "paying it forward" if daily exercise isn't already in your daily schedule. How would you feel if you looked great in a sleeveless top at age 60, could race up a set of stairs at 65, or shop and put away your own groceries at 70? Integrating fitness into your life now delivers immediate and future results. Simply adding a daily walk will help you on your way!

Take *Action* #10: Plan Your Health Goals

Take five minutes to start planning your critical life project and entitle it: "My Health." Want to be a zoomer boomer, a go-getter who lives life to the fullest? Include a strategy for retirement *fitness*. It's just as important as your 401K, social security, and pension plan. Like any other plan, you will check your milestones and revise. Then you get to execute and evaluate the plan. Using your project management skills to help change your life now will help you lead a fitter, fuller, and healthier life, even when every day is Saturday.

Jot down fitness and health goals for every decade of your life going forward:

Year:

_____

Year:

_____

Year:

_____

Year:

_____

Look at these goals often, to be certain you are engaged in the physical activities that will help support you.

Exercise Excuse #7:
"I'm too old to start now."

Nice try. I might surprise you here, but the reality is that much of what we consider normal aging is due to physical inactivity. Only 15-20% of disease is to due to hereditary factors. This leaves much of our aging experience up to us. As we age, we can become "elderly," or choose to create another label: "wellderly." I know people in each of these categories. Which sounds better to you?

The fitness fountain of youth

Because exercise is so customizable and adaptable to most any age, I call it the fountain of youth. In fact, many older clients come to me because they want to remain independent as they grow older. Being functionally fit allows older adults to stay in their homes and direct their own lives, steering clear of the "disability zone" for years longer than those who don't make exercise a daily focus.

Long-standing research demonstrates that the introduction of even a modest strength training regime at any age improves fitness levels. Even 90-year-old nursing home residents can become stronger. Some even walk after being confined to a wheelchair! I have a colleague who teaches yoga-in-a-chair for acute-care residents. They love it! Since one of the top five reasons older folks are admitted to the hospital is due to falls, including stability and flexibility exercises and yoga-like stretches in your fitness plan diminishes that fear and chance of falling.

Isn't independence important to you? I thought so.

Younger next year

In their book, *Younger Next Year*, Henry S. Lodge, MD, and his 70-year-old patient, Chris Crowley, show you how you can be functionally younger for years after your 50th birthday, and retain much of your physical health well into your eighties. They explain that although Americans expect to "get old and die" most of us will unfortunately "get old and live."

Dr. Lodge suggests, "Aerobic exercise saves your life; strength training makes it worth living." "Old" can be a relative term and. I agree! He implores you to make exercise a "job"—an activity that you do right now (whether or not you are in retirement years) and beyond to stem the tide of lifestyle-related diseases and ailments.

Successtimonial: My body just got rusty

Julie, a 68-year-old homemaker recently phoned me and asked about my fitness coaching services. She said she felt her body had "rusted" and she was quickly becoming unable to get up and down the stairs without body aches, but she was uncertain if she was too old to do something about it. I bet you can guess my response.

Now, after a few months focusing on walking and improving her strength and flexibility, Julie is easily able to get down and play on the floor with her grandchildren and get up without assistance. Her new goal is one millions of people can relate to: to be "sleeveless by summer," and I have no doubt that she will reach it.

You are as young as your body and mind feel

The classic adage "You are only as young as you feel" is a great mantra for everyone. Get up and claim fitness for yourself and you will see and feel the difference.

A growing body of research shows the benefits of exercise are just as significant for those in their 70s and beyond as for younger people, according to Duke University Medical Center researchers. They believe regular exercise can in fact slow or even reverse some of the effects of aging that were once thought to be inevitable.

James Blumenthal, PhD, Duke University professor of medical psychology reports: "Exercise improves psychological functioning, in terms of reducing symptoms of distress, anxiety, and depression, In addition, exercise has been shown to improve self-esteem and self-confidence."

He goes on to explain, "We also see clear benefits of exercise on physical functioning. It reduces the risk for cardiovascular disease, lowers cholesterol, builds bone density, and lowers the risk of osteoporosis. There's a suggestion that it lowers blood pressure, and even data to suggest that the risk of having gallstones is reduced with exercise."

An important insight from this study is that the physical activity you choose doesn't have to be intensive to reap important health benefits.

Blumenthal states: "You don't need to run a marathon. You'll see benefits from walking, biking, and other simple activities."

Like most Americans, older folks are simply not getting enough exercise. Blumenthal said the current recommendation is to try and get at least some aerobic exercise every day or almost every day. He says 30 minutes a day, five days a week, is optimal.

Would you like to lower your health care costs? Research shows that exercise can help. Regular physical activity can facilitate weight loss and weight management and can help regulate blood sugar levels to control Type 2 diabetes. Obesity and diabetes are two of America's most serious public health problems, reports Blumenthal.

"It's never too late to start exercising," he said. "Exercise can help an older person improve their physical fitness, muscle strength, and aerobic capacity, as well as their mood and cognitive abilities. There was a belief a number of years ago that beyond a certain age, people wouldn't get the same benefits from exercise as a younger person would. Now we know that's not the case."

Take *Action* #11: Pick Three Fitness Goals

No matter how old you are, jot down three things you would like to accomplish by this time next year (i.e., learn to do a flip turn in the pool, walk up and down three flights of stairs without having to rest on each landing, hold your twin grandbabies one in each arm, or walk from the parking lot to the water's edge at the beach). Think functionally what body mechanics would be necessary (stamina to walk or strong arms and shoulders to hold the babies) and find modest exercises that can help you get there. Start with slow, steady, and controlled movements, a few at a time. As you gain strength, your body will tell you when to make the exercises a bit harder, or you can work with a fitness professional who can be your expert guide.

1. ————————————————————————————

2. ————————————————————————————

3. ————————————————————————————

Exercise Excuse #6:

"I tried and I failed in the past."

"Never confuse a single defeat with a final defeat."
—F. Scott Fitzgerald

Let's say the past is past. You can't drive your car forward looking in the rearview mirror. Let's agree to look forward, not back. Fair?

Take *Action* #12: Look Back to Move Forward

Before we leave the past entirely, jot down three reasons why you believe you failed in your previous attempts to exercise. Please be honest. I am not looking over your shoulder!

I failed in my previous attempts to exercise because:

1. _____

_____

2. _____

_____

3. _____

_____

I have encountered hundreds of people who have "tried and failed in the past." Here are the two top reasons people fail in their quest for fitness:

1. **Setting the bar too high.**

     Most of my clients have begun a new program and set unreachable goals, such as "I'll work out an hour every day!" "I'll go to the gym six days a week!" or "I'll always take the stairs at work!"

     In the warm-up section of this book, we talked about black-or-white thinking. Let's apply that learning here. What happens when you set the bar too high and don't quite make it or when life gets in the way of your newfound commitment? Do you feel bad? Do you wonder "what's the use?" If so, it's inevitable that your resolve will crumble.

     Sound familiar? Good, let go of the guilt . . .

     This time, why not do what I ask my clients to do? Start slowly. Commit to do less than what you are capable of. How about 10 or 15 minutes of exercise every other day? Go to the gym two times a week or take the stairs at work on even-numbered days? It may not seem like enough, but it's a great start.

     This approach leads to more success, and guess what? You may even exceed your initial goals. WOW! That's a nice feeling, isn't it? You get to pat yourself on the back! "Atta boy/girl!" Time to celebrate.

2. Letting the past dictate your future.

Think about something in your past that you tried several times. You kept at it, perhaps after failing in the beginning. The old "one step forward and two steps back" tango.

A common experience might be learning to ride a bicycle, ski, or drive the lawn tractor. Maybe your bike experience went a bit like this: First you had a tricycle that required very little balance or skill. You were a terror on it! Then you got that big boy/girl bike with those helpful training wheels, you took to it easily and had tons of fun!

Then came "The Day." The training wheels came off and your parents were ready with the camera. Half a revolution of the pedals and down you went. Your knees were scraped and your ego bruised. But your parents were, for some reason, clapping and cheering. They encouraged you. "Eddie that was great! You're almost there! Just a few more tries and you'll be a pro!" And guess what? You were!

So, let's not label yourself a fitness loser, okay? This fitness thing is something you can do. Learn from your past experiences by reevaluating what went wrong and altering it this time around.

- Did you try to do too much too quickly? Ouch! That can hurt! This is where I see so much failure and it's simply not necessary. In fitness, you don't have to start big, you just have to start and be consistent.
- Did you have some false starts and side steps? Change is not always a linear process. Sometimes you need to stop

and shout "do over!" It worked when you were a child and it can work today.

- Did you lose sight of *you* in your daily schedule? Making time for yourself is the best way to live a full, productive, and happy life. You are special and deserve your own attention. Setting time for fitness is important self-care.

Remember, you can do it! You can't see right away when your cholesterol is lowering or your blood pressure is becoming regulated, but that doesn't mean it isn't happening. A longer, healthier life is definitely worth the effort.

Successtimonial: Less is more

Charles was a busy doctor who had recently lost 25 pounds and wanted to become more competitive in tennis. In our first meeting, I learned that except for one weekly doubles tennis match he was not doing any exercise. He balked at my suggestion of starting with and committing to what he called a "measly" 20 minutes of treadmill walking three times a week. He was adamant that he would be on his treadmill a minimum of 30 minutes daily; however, he trusted my judgment and vowed to give this less challenging workout a try. Before our next session, I received an e-mail from Charles that his partner had been called away on a family emergency and he had to see double the number of patients, but was still able to squeeze in the 20 minutes of walking we agreed upon. His last lines were: "I realized that I was a winner even when my schedule got upended. I feel great about what I am accomplishing!"

And so will you.

Exercise Excuse #5:

"Exercise is boring. It's too hard. I hate it."

"When you come right down to it, the secret of having it all is loving it all."
—Dr. Joyce Brothers

WOW! That's a mouthful of complaints I hear frequently.

In my business, these are some of the most challenging client excuses. My mother always said, "Only the boring are bored." Thanks, Mom. Boredom is a funny thing; it's a decision that you make based on a perception, a type of self-fulfilling prophecy and unlike other excuses. So what makes exercise boring, too hard, or not fun? You do.

Granted, some exercise movements are repetitive and tedious. For you scientific types, this exercise equation might look like:

Exercise = repetition
Repetition = boring
Therefore, exercise = boring

Add in isolation, and I can see how some people really hate it. The poor treadmill is even maligned as the definition of going nowhere. You may lament, "How can I get and stay motivated about going nowhere?"

The way I look at it, the key is to participate in activities that you enjoy and with people you like. Remember that pain/pleasure theory? Making exercise interesting, doable, and fun can depend on your current health condition(s) and your personality. Maybe you are gregarious or fiercely independent; it all impacts your success when it comes to exercise. Getting encouragement and special attention can help the obese, medically challenged, or fledgling exercisers learn how to safely get started.

You can't get motivated to exercise?

Is it that you can't get started or that you have trouble staying on your path? What if you are invited to your high school reunion or the wedding of your best friend's daughter? Does that motivate you? These events, including the infamous New Year's resolution, are *external*, harnessing the power of something outside of yourself to get you moving. This can work, but as we have painfully experienced, only for the short term. What if you don't have that compelling event on your calendar?

Why not create a reason based on your own goals: bathing suit season, wearing your favorite jeans, or beginning to date again.

You may start an exercise program because of an external event or goal, but the key to maintaining your focus and living a fit life is the commitment to continue well after the excitement of that event has passed. External motivation can jump start you, but it won't keep you on your path.

I know my clients have leaped over this hurdle when they are motivated by *internal* forces; having more energy and enthusiasm, liking themselves more, and being healthier than in the past. It's a subtle shift, but when they report feeling odd if they don't exercise, it's a clear intention for a lifelong commitment and certainly something to celebrate!

There really is no finish line in fitness. It's a lifestyle. It's true that exercise sounds great right up till the moment you have to do it. The idea itself can be daunting. You might be reading this and think, "I can't even get jazzed to get out of my chair, how can I ever get motivated to sweat, lift a weight, and maybe deal with an occasional sore muscle or two most days of the week?" Ugh!

Try naming your reason for exercising. It might be size 10 jeans, holding your new granddaughter, or 120/80 blood pressure.

Sometimes it's not easy to make an important lifestyle change, even when people's lives are threatened. It's a common scenario: A cardiac patient arrives at the hospital on a stretcher after experiencing a heart attack. After the immediate danger is averted (by various scary medical interventions), the patient is given a long list of changes they must make to decrease the chances of a return trip.

You may think "Of course they will change their life. There is big motivation here!" And, most people do, while being closely supervised during cardiac recovery. Unfortunately, research has proven over and over that many patients slip back into their normal routine and start the cycle all over again.

Why not impress yourself?

Don't be frustrated. Exercise doesn't have to be hard. Why not look at increased physical activity as a few small changes that you do every day? Identify small, totally accomplishable goals. Walk to your mailbox to get the mail instead of driving there, use the restroom farthest away from your office, walk up and down each grocery aisle before checking out. Starting with small activities gives you little successes that motivate you forward to larger goals. Ideas like these have worked for many of my clients and they can work for you too.

What other ideas can you think of for your particular circumstances? Jot them down; you'll need them for the next Take Action assignment. Use the assignments in previous chapters to remind yourself of the behaviors and the affirmations I provide later in this book to help keep you on target.

Take *Action* #13: Create Your Health Benefits List

After a few weeks of minor changes, set 10 minutes aside to review your progress. Write down how you are feeling, listing all the positive benefits that moving more has on your life. We'll call it *Your Health Benefits List*. It's so critical to your positive behavior shift I want you to write it down. Don't discount being able to walk up stairs without being winded, stand up from your chair without relying on the arms, or bending over without discomfort. It's all very significant.

What? You don't think so? Why is it that as an adult you don't acknowledge the small, positive shifts in your fitness level; improvements that you would applaud in your best friend but minimize in yourself? It's puzzling for certain. You now have permission to act like a child again and impress yourself!

Don't forget to post your benefits list (it will grow longer each week) in a place you'll see regularly. It will remind you *why* you are exercising. After a few months of consistent effort, you will feel odd if you don't move, the true test that you have altered your behavior and made internal cues to motivate your daily activity. And, that is truly impressive!

My Health Benefits List
What differences do I feel? Share the self love!

_____

_____

_____

_____

Take *Action* #14: Find Your Exercise Personality

Take this exercise personality test by selecting the option that is most true for you:

1. I work out (or want to work out) because:
   a. I want to look better and/or lose weight.
   b. I want to clear my head and/or reduce stress.
   c. I love to move and be active.
2. I get a lot of joy from:
   a. Spending time with the people I love.
   b. Working toward a goal or a dream.
   c. Pushing myself to my physical limits.
3. I'd rather be:
   a. Talking on the phone with a good friend.
   b. Working on a project or furthering my career.
   c. Doing my favorite sport or activity.

If you answered:

<u>Mostly A's:</u> You are people-oriented and may avoid gyms if you perceive them as unattractive or impersonal places. You want to find something fun, so think about joining a team sport or hiking group, or organize some friends to exercise with.

<u>Mostly B's:</u> You are goal-oriented and on a mission! You may do your best with a time-efficient video workout, lunch-time class, or a trainer who can give you specific routines for home use. Sticking

to your plan is imperative for you, because you will be revved up by your results.

<u>Mostly C's:</u> You are action-oriented and rarely sit still. A group class where the instructor sets the pace and doesn't allow you to skip the warm-up or run out early will keep you engaged. A varied selection of activities will keep you interested and those that connect your mind and body, such as yoga or tai chi would be excellent exercise choices.

So, remind me . . . what's tiresome, boring, or dull about feeling great, looking fabulous, and—most of all—being happy with yourself?

Successtimonial: Make exercise palatable

Ann doesn't complain much about walking on the beach, but frequently and vehemently states how *boring* the treadmill, elliptical, and even the bike are. She claimed that even watching TV or listening to music didn't do much to improve the tedium. We came up with an idea, based on her love of variety and Chinese food, to create a pu pu platter of cardiovascular exercise: 10 minutes on the treadmill, 10 minutes on the elliptical, and, you get the idea, 10 minutes on the bike. Ann says "I get a full 30 minutes of heart-healthy exercise without wanting to scream!" Use this unique fitness menu to your advantage. Bon Appetit!

Exercise Excuse #4:

"I have health problems/old injuries."

"It is better to burn out than it is to rust."
—Neil Young

You may have collected health problems or injuries like some people collect baseball memorabilia. Many folks believe that their physical or medical issues give them a free pass when it comes to fitness. If that's what you choose to believe, no one will be able to dissuade you. However, if you are open to considering where you are today in relation to your fitness goals, and have decided you want to improve, this is the right chapter for you!

Take *Action* #15: What *Can* You Do?

Forget about what you cannot do because of a bum knee, arthritis, cancer, etc., and brainstorm all the activities, exercises, or sports that you *can* do. Don't disregard the ones you don't like; just note what you are physically able to do. You can discard items from the list later.

Sample List of Activities:

Ballroom dance	Biking
Tennis	Skiing

Swimming	Country line dancing
Bowling	Yoga
Walking	Pilates
Gardening	Running
Nordic pole walking	Stair climbing/stepping
Weightlifting	Irish dancing
Water aerobics	Wheelchair/chair yoga

See? You've realized there are actions your body can still do! Now, select three of those activities/sports or fun movements and commit to doing one of them this week. Add the second in week two, and the third in week three. Don't forget to start slow, as pushing yourself too fast will most certainly lead to muscle soreness, which can begin the cycle of feeling like every workout is the first one—and that's no fun!

Successtimonial: Hey! I can do it!

Paul began working with me with a long list of his "can't dos" which included running, stair climbing, and heavy lifting due to a work-related back injury that had plagued him for years.

He did this assignment and selected bike riding, walking the dog, and ballroom dancing as three activities that he could physically do and actually thought he might enjoy. The first week he rode a recumbent bike (the kind that you sit back in vs. an upright bike) for 15 minutes on three days. The second week he rode his bike twice and walked the dog for half an hour. The third week, he rode his bike twice, walked the dog for half an hour, and took his first ballroom dance class.

Did I tell you that Paul is 72 years old? Paul is now riding his bike most days, walking his pooch three times a week (the dog and Paul have both lost weight), and he is his dance instructor's favorite student.

Exercise benefits for America's top five diseases

According to many top health organizations, including the Mayo Clinic and the National Institutes of Health, almost anyone can do some type of physical activity, even folks with conditions such as diabetes, cancer, heart disease, arthritis, and obesity. In fact, research continues to reveal that exercise may help these diseases and other medical conditions.

Here are some of the reported benefits of exercise for America's top five disease conditions:

Diabetes

Exercise can be extremely effective in helping to manage both Type I and Type II diabetes, in addition to assisting with insulin-resistance issues. Exercise can reduce your need for glucose-lowering medication, maintain healthy circulation in your arms and legs, improve your cardiovascular health, and keep your weight in check.

If you are new to the idea, wear comfortable sneakers and try a conservative walking program twice a week, increasing the frequency (additional times per week), intensity (perhaps walking up a hill or two), and time (longer walks). Include gentle yoga postures such as "mountain" (standing straight with both feet flat and grounded, arms up alongside your head) and "chair" (arms up, both legs bent, buttocks slightly lowered, like sitting), along with deep breathing to help create a calm feeling.

Cancer

In the past, people with serious chronic diseases such as cancer have been advised by their doctors to avoid physical activity and increase rest. In the case of recent surgery, or if exercise causes rapid heart rate, dizziness, or severe pain this may still be the case. However, the American Cancer Society advocates that for many cancer patients, exercise is beneficial. The ACS studies consistently list these three benefits of exercise:

- Improved physical fitness.
- Higher self-esteem.
- Lower levels of anxiety, depression, and fatigue.

A cancer diagnosis and ensuing chemotherapy or radiation treatments can leave you depressed, tired, and lethargic. However, there are certified cancer exercise trainers (I am proud to be one) who help patients with specialized exercise programs. What we now know is that exercise not only engages your body but your mind as well. It can offer you an improved sense of well-being and significantly decrease the fatigue and anxiety that accompanies cancer treatments. Exercise has also been proven to help decrease the chance of a recurrence for many cancers.

Heart Disease

Aerobic exercise is well documented as a critical component in a heart healthy life and as a therapy for those diagnosed with heart disease. Scottish scientists reported in the *Journal of the American College of Cardiology* that a single session of exercise improved the health of blood vessels and reduced lipid levels in men. Aerobic exercise, also known as cardiovascular exercise, conditions the heart and lungs by increasing the oxygen available to the body and enabling the heart to use oxygen more efficiently.

Arthritis

Arthritis Today magazine often receives letters from readers who say they want to work out, but find it hard to get out of their chair or walk across the room, let alone jog around the block. If this sounds like you, there's good news. Exercises can be done sitting in a supportive chair, your favorite recliner, or even a wheelchair.

Successtimonial: Finding the right exercise for you

Rhonda is a 67-year-old arthritis sufferer who says there have been many days when she couldn't stand up or walk across a room. "But even when I couldn't get up out of the chair, I could still move," she said. In her chair, she does shoulder rolls, leg lifts with light ankle weights, and arm raises. Rhonda also uses a stationary bike, water exercises, and resistance bands. Instead of sapping your energy, exercise will limber and lubricate your painful joints.

Obesity

One out of three Americans is obese. Exercise intervention can be an effective option along with a balanced food plan to provide the daily caloric deficit that leads to weight loss. Exercise as therapy includes the use of aerobic exercise (such as dancing, brisk walking, cycling, and swimming), beginning slowly and gradually increasing intensity. For individuals new to exercise, it's critical to select enjoyable activities that can be scheduled into a regular routine.

I hope you see your capabilities in a different way now, with more of a "can do" attitude. There is power in a decision followed by the action to make something happen.

Congratulations for rethinking your situation and moving past your roadblocks!

Exercise Excuse #3:

"I'm too fat and out of shape."

"People become really quite remarkable when they start thinking that they can do things. When they believe in themselves they have the first secret to success."
—Norman Vincent Peale

You may be reading through this book, get to this chapter and see yourself, knowing in your heart that your weight is spinning out of control and your body is deconditioned. If you relate to this excuse, hurray! You are still with me. Allow me to pick up my cheerleader pom poms and bust through this excuse right now.

Maybe you have struggled with your weight all your life, or maybe it's a new and unfamiliar feeling. Maybe your weight is stable, but through the years you have noticed your energy decreasing, struggling to climb stairs, bend, stretch, or lift boxes.

I like to say, "If not now, when?" As your personal fitness motivator, I am belting out a cheer for you to take one step in the direction of improved health. You've learned that small steps will deliver great rewards and almost everyone, at any age, size, or health situation can and should exercise.

The fitness latte factor

David Bach, finance wizard and popular author made the phrase "The Latte Factor®" very famous. In his books, the latte factor is used to illustrate that seemingly insignificant amounts of money, when saved regularly and over time, will grow into a significant sum. I like to apply his theory in this way: seemingly insignificant physical activities, done consistently, will deliver noticeable health and fitness benefits.

Successtimonial: Small steps, great rewards

Leslie is a lovely woman who was obese and suffering from a bad back, knee pain, and flat feet when we met. Her doctor had even authorized a handicapped pass so she could park her car close to the door at work.

In our initial conversations, Leslie indicated that there was very little in the way of movement that she could accomplish. This was a big challenge, but developing creative strategies is what I do. So I took some time to carefully study what Leslie did every day and how she might be able to move more in her normal activities. What I came up with was something Leslie could accomplish daily.

Her assignment was to walk around her car with her hand supporting her along the way each and every time she got in to drive anywhere. Okay, her neighbors thought there was something a bit weird happening in the driveway across the street, but Leslie agreed to this idea and in a few days was walking three times around her car before driving away. Her kids, not wanting to be left out, also got in on the fun.

Leslie realized that starting with something she could accomplish in her personal situation was the way she could begin to get fit. A year after that very modest consistent daily activity, additional attention to her eating plan, and putting herself first, she was walking on a treadmill most days and had lost more than 100 pounds. She happily gave up her handicapped parking pass in celebration.

The cool thing is that the heavier and more out of shape you are, the greater the initial benefits will be, even when your efforts are conservative and seemingly insignificant. So, what's your excuse?

Talk nice to yourself

I am guessing that you may encounter a few moments of frustration, disappointment, and overwhelm while you are trying this new, active life. Don't give up! Please consider the use of positive affirmations to help you. Here are a few that my clients have relied on to put one foot in front of the other, literally:

- Every step I take leads me to a fitter, healthier life.
- I am capable of positive changes today.
- Nothing tastes as good as fit and healthy feels.
- I am stronger and more vigorous today.
- I am an active, energetic, joyful person.

Take *Action* #16: Make Movement a Game

Start moving. Sounds easy, huh? Well, you may not think it's all that simple. Games are fun, so how about making a game out of it?

Try these ideas or create your own:

1. Don't sit down at the computer or TV until you have walked around the inside of your home, climbed one flight of stairs, or lifted some 1-lb. soup cans 10 times. Every time you get up from the seat, repeat or select another activity.

2. Get up 30 minutes earlier twice a week (increase as you get fitter), don your outdoor gear and sneakers, and take a quiet walk around the block (or the perimeter of your home). You can go slowly; there's no need to make it a power walk, especially at first. Think positive thoughts about yourself.

3. Look in the mirror daily and state clearly and confidently: "I am hot and awesome" and/or "I love you!" Or "I am one of God's unique and beautiful creations" Yes, it seems silly, but with the thousands of not nice messages you speak/think about your body, at least introduce one affirming statement daily.

Talk nice to yourself, support your efforts and see how your body makes you proud!

Exercise Excuse #2:

"I am just too tired, period."

"I bless my body with loving exercise. It revitalizes me inside and out."
—Louise Hay

Uh oh, I can almost see your exhausted expression, slumped shoulders, and dragging feet! Feeling like this is common with our frantic daily pace, so don't fret. However, this is another great excuse that holds you back from being the fabulously fit person you can be.

You may be best friends with the sisters that represent this excuse; I call them Sedentary and Lethargy. You are working more, you are sleeping less, you are not exercising. Meet Sedentary. Add eating at the wrong times, perhaps the wrong foods, and definitely on the run. You are exhausted, physically and mentally. Enter Lethargy. Okay, that's reality.

Let's focus more on how to recharge your personal batteries and sustain zest for your marvelous life. In the warm-up chapter we talked about exercise as it truly is; fueling your own personal energy plant. Yes, it does take some stored up energy to get the plant going. Everything important takes a bit of work, right? But once the plant is operating, it delivers more energy. Simply said, the more you move, the more energy you have. It's Newton's First Law of Motion:

> ! | *An object at rest tends to stay at rest and an object in motion tends to stay in motion.*

Take *Action* #17: M O V E!

The next time you think you are just too exhausted to do one more thing, don't succumb to a nap, reach for the coffee cup, or unwrap that candy bar. Both caffeine and sugar will provide a short burst of energy, but that the boost is short-lived. Think instead of this four letter word: M O V E.

Have that exercise or dance video queued up and ready to go. Put on your favorite music and give yourself three minutes to move. That's all. Walk, dance, march in place, anything that gets your legs and arms moving. At the three-minute mark, you have permission to stop moving, or like my clients love to breathlessly and joyfully declare, *keep moving!*

Hey, you might even feel good enough to continue your choice of movement for a few more minutes. Then I want you to tune into your body and answer these questions:

1. How do I feel?
2. Am I smiling/laughing?
3. Am I breathing a bit harder?

4. Can I continue this activity for a few more minutes if it extends my life?
5. Am I having fun yet?

That's how easy it can be to pump up the power in your life. Keep it up and you and everyone around you will notice the smile on your face, your lilting step, and shoulders back, chin-up approach to life.

Let's escort Sedentary and Lethargy to the door because you are so over this excuse.

Successtimonial: Mommy movement

Mary was a young mom of three, including a special-needs child whose care took all of her waking and sleeping hours. She knew in her logical mind that exercise was lacking in her life, but her body felt way too tired to do anything about it. She wanted to know she'd feel the difference after she exercised—before she tried it.

And that's the trick. Knowing with certainty that you will feel more energized, more alive, and essentially happier after you move—which you cannot prove until you move! It's a catch 22.

Mary allowed herself four weeks to do things differently and to see what happened. Within two weeks she was smiling more, enjoying her children, and "feeling 10 years younger." Two years after starting her modest movement increase, Mary leads a mommy and me yoga class for developmentally challenged children.

! | *Act and then you will feel. If you __wait__ to feel, you will never __act__.*

Exercise boosts energy better than stimulants

New research from the University of Georgia suggests that regular exercise can increase energy levels even in the most fatigued individuals. Exercise has been proven to be a powerful "drug," boosting the happy chemicals in the brain. It may seem counter-intuitive, but researchers say expending energy by engaging in regular exercise may pay off with increased energy in the long run.

"A lot of times when people are fatigued, the last thing they want to do is exercise," says researcher Patrick O'Connor, PhD, codirector of the University of Georgia exercise psychology laboratory in Athens, Ga., in a news release. "But if you're physically inactive and fatigued, being just a bit more active will help."

"We live in a society where people are always looking for the next sports drink, energy bar, or cup of coffee that will give them the extra edge to get through the day," says researcher Tim Puetz, PhD, also of UGA. "But it may be that lacing up your tennis shoes and getting out and doing some physical activity every morning can provide that spark of energy that people are looking for."

Sedentary people reduce fatigue with exercise

Studies have actually quantified the hypothesis that sedentary people who start a regular exercise program experience an increase in energy levels. A study published in *Psychological Bulletin* reported it's researchers analyzed 70 studies on exercise and fatigue involving more than 6,800 people.

"More than 90% of the studies showed the same thing: Sedentary people who completed a regular exercise program affirmed that fatigue decreased compared to groups that did not exercise," says O'Connor. "It's a very consistent effect."

Take *Action* #18: Fatigue Busting 101

1. Rate your level of fatigue at the beginning, middle, and end of each day on a scale of 1-10 (1 means "I am not tired," 10 means "I am dead on my feet").
2. Determine during which timeframe you are *most* fatigued.
3. During that time, take a brisk walk, a brief jog, or climb a flight of stairs. Try 3-5 minutes. You can do this whether you are at the office or at home.
4. Retest your fatigue level after this burst of activity.
5. Give yourself a gold star. You did great!
6. After a week of this behavior, celebrate again. Who thought this fitness stuff could be such fun and so empowering?
7. Repeat, have fun, add more minutes, have fun, add different activities, celebrate. You get the idea.

Exercise Excuse #1:

"I simply don't have the time."

"Life all comes down to a few moments. This is one of them."
—Bud Fox (from the movie *Wall Street*)

Here we are, at the top of the list, to the excuse that more than 40% of Americans said was the main reason they crossed exercising off their list.

You are busy! Busy, *busy,* **BUSY!** With your job, your family, and the digital tether that follows you everywhere. Time is the easiest cop-out for not exercising. Busy mom? Cube dweller? Many professions and avocations are more than an overtime job, they're a lifetime commitment. "No time" is a justification that sounds good, but it simply doesn't fly if you are honest with yourself.

Everyone has the same 1,440 minutes in each and every day, and I bet you can name at least three busy people who get everything, including their workout, done. What most successful people know is putting themselves and their health first allows them to be their best—in the boardroom and beyond.

Exercise is self-care of the highest degree. Put yourself on your daily to-do list, on the first line, in pen. Don't hit the Delete key on your time. YOU DESERVE IT!

I like to appeal to my logical readers with this equation:

If exercise = self-care
And self-care = increased capacity
Then exercise = increased capacity

Isn't that what everyone wants? Increased capacity to have fun, make money, live, and love? Since I know right now (I peeked at your personal time journal) that your schedule isn't crammed with high-value physical activity every minute you are awake, you simply must make the time to exercise. You might not have 30 solid minutes or more to devote daily to exercise, but you certainly have 10 or 15 minutes here and there to give yourself the gift of improved health and fitness. Let's call it a Fitness Break.

Remember what we discussed in the warm-up chapter? When something is very important to you, you make it happen. Since your future health depends on your current choices and activities, each day presents many opportunities to get up, move, and improve.

Take short fitness activity breaks during your normal day so you don't feel pressured to take long amounts of time out of your schedule. Do more when you can and when you are feeling exceptionally sassy. I recommend that you find a way to exercise the first thing in the morning. It gets your day started in a positive, self-affirming way. Even 15 minutes of yoga before your shower works since later in the day, even the best-intentioned individual can get side-tracked, leaving fitness in the day's ashes.

Take *Action* #19: Keep a Fitness Calendar

Keep a calendar of your fitness breaks so you can track your progress. Every 10-15 minutes of stretching, lifting, or walking gets you credit. At the end of the day, give yourself a grade, just like your childhood report cards.

Here's your scale:
A = Active
B = Basic
C = Couch (like couch potato)

Award yourself an "A" if your day had some structured exercise time such as time on the treadmill, yoga class, or a gym visit, along with two or more Fitness Breaks. Add parking farther away from the office, walking to your colleagues' office vs. e-mailing, walking to the furthest restroom from you, and other ways to move more. Schedule your exercise time. Even if you keep this appointment 50% of the time, it's probably 100% more than you were doing before.

You earn a "B" if your day didn't have any structure exercise, but you get credit for one or two Fitness Breaks and the effort you demonstrated by walking around the perimeter of the grocery store, pacing while on the phone, or lifting soup or trash cans.

You get a "C" if you find your day was spent sitting in the car/train/plane, in front of your computer, or in meetings. No Fitness

Breaks or extra effort was put forth to move and you didn't do any structured exercise.

Now, at the end of the week, average your grade and see how you did. Evaluate your progress and learn from the past week. Next week you can do better! Remember, no one will see these grades but you. However, please share them with your fitness professional if you are working with one. Don't forget to plan a backup schedule for when you are on vacation, a business trip, or just pressed for time.

Remember, life happens. It's not always black or white. Be ready with alternatives, and if you miss a workout, practice kind self-forgiveness. If you need to start your fitness program over again, call a "do over," pick up where you left off, and build up again.

Final Thoughts

It has been my privilege to share my thoughts with you.

You are a unique, loving, and worthy individual who deserves to live your best life *ever*. You have the power in this moment to change the way you think about where you are heading with your health and fitness and do something *awesome* about it.

You can reshape your world starting now and claim a fit, healthy life as your own.

I called them exercise excuses, but now you see what they really are: fitness triumphs just waiting to bust out and happen.

"Great things are not done by impulse, but by a series of small things brought together."
—Vincent van Gogh

Get up, take those first steps, and do great things. For you. Let me know how things are going on Facebook, Twitter, or my blog.

How to Choose a Personal Trainer

It seems all the celebrities have them. Elite athletes have them. Should *you* have a personal trainer?

I am often asked about how to decide whether to work with a personal trainer and how to find one that is right for you. Here are some ideas.

Every American knows that exercise is the answer to many health-related problems. A regular exercise routine can help reduce health risks such as diabetes, heart disease, and cancer. You can't go a day without being bombarded with statistics concerning obesity and how inactive, lethargic, and unhealthy our society is. It's estimated that more than 85% of disease is lifestyle-related, but most people lack the motivation to increase activity and move consistently. When a doctor tells them to "lose weight and exercise," most people literally throw up their hands in frustration. "When? How? Where? Why bother?"

That's where a personal trainer can help with motivation, education, and more. A trainer is an experienced educator, professional coach, and cheerleader who will customize a program for you that works toward your specific goals and incorporates your lifestyle. They will consider your interests along with understanding and respecting any limitations you may have. Some people use a personal trainer several times a week in their home, office, or gym. Others have them set up an initial program and then check in on a sporadic basis to get feedback, monitor progress, and update programs. Most fitness centers also make personal training available to their members.

People ask me why they should consider engaging a personal trainer. As I see it, if you were interested in learning to play the piano, wouldn't you locate an instructor who is an expert? If you wanted to learn how to cook French cuisine, wouldn't learning from an experienced chef make sense? Think of a trainer as a coach and mentor whose job it is to help you improve your health and physical condition.

Your personal trainer will:
- Assess your current physical condition and become part of your personal circle of care along with your physicians, physical therapist, chiropractor, etc.
- Craft a specific program for you, taking into consideration your current physical condition and any medical conditions such as diabetes, heart disease, cancer, arthritis, and obesity.
- Provide one-on-one supervision, making sure you use proper form and technique so you get the most from your time and effort with decreased chance of injury.
- Assure that you address all aspects of fitness, including cardiovascular activity, strength training, balance, stretching, and flexibility as appropriate.
- Help you overcome roadblocks and challenges, truly supporting you toward becoming your personal best.

Finding a personal trainer is fairly easy. Finding the right trainer for you may take a bit of time and effort, but will be well worth it.

Inquire at your local health club or chamber of commerce, check the local newspaper, telephone book, or the Internet. Don't forget to ask your friends and colleagues. You might be surprised at how many people are already working with a trainer.

Criteria for interviewing and selecting a personal trainer:
- Ask about national certification and current CPR certification. Professional trainers must pass a series of tests and continuing education credits to maintain their certification.
- Ask about their experience. Everyone is different, with different goals, interests, and challenges. Find a trainer that can offer what you need.
- Ask for client references—one of the best ways to gauge if the trainer is right for you.
- Confirm that the trainer will keep records and is willing to communicate with your doctor or physical therapist if needed.
- Ask about their liability insurance, cancellation policies, and inquire about the approximate length of a session.
- Confirm fees and any package pricing in advance. Trainer fees can vary greatly depending on your location, the trainers experience and specialty expertise. Many trainers offer series pricing, tandem rates (1 trainer and 2 clients at the same time), and other creative budgeting options.

And, throughout the training relationship ask yourself:
- Do you still like your trainer?
- Do they educate you and communicate well?
- Do you have confidence in their ability?

- Do they demonstrate commitment to your goals?
- Does your relationship build *your* confidence?

Whether you are young, retired, healthy, or health-compromised, one of the most effective ways to get started, add variety, or shake up your fitness program is to have a personal trainer guide the way. Have fun!

About the Author

Setting new trends in training and motivation, personal trainer, cancer trainer, wellness educator and active lifestyle coach, Linda Gottlieb has had an extensive career in the fitness industry. She has developed and presented hundreds of exercise/wellness classes, has been director of a 30,000 square foot, full service health club and has managed fitness facility projects for luxury hotels.

Along with traditional in-home personal fitness training, Linda specializes in individualized telephone/email coaching, addressing the long neglected busy, working professionals who are either uncomfortable with or don't have the time to commit to conventional personal training programs.

In 2007, she launched FitChicks, a monthly support group with workshops held in Shelton, CT to help women take small steps to a fitter, healthier life.

Ms. Gottlieb's undergraduate degree in Psychology, along with her Masters degree in Instructional Design prepare her to successfully interpret motivation of her clients, work through roadblocks and stages of behavioral change. She also excels at presenting fitness and active lifestyle theory and methodologies in an easy to understand manner, engaging her clients at all levels.

Linda received the Presidential Sports Award in 1988 and 2003, multiple industry certifications from IDEA, ACE, and AFAA, and is a member of The American Institute of Fitness Educators, The Association of Fitness by Phone® Coaches and Reebok Instructor Alliance. She holds current Adult CPR certification from the American Red Cross and is the first nationally certified Cooper Institute Active Living Every Day behavior change program facilitator in the state of Connecticut.

Linda is on the staff of Yale University as Cancer Exercise Trainer for exercise trials studying the benefits of increased physical activity in cancer patients and survivors.

Ms. Gottlieb is a frequent speaker, championing daily fitness activity, the connection between food and mood, and realistic and positive perceptions of an individual's body image. In addition to her first book, ***No Ifs, Ands, or Butts: How to Turn the Top 10 Exercise Excuses into Fitness Triumphs***, she also supports her clients with a monthly Optimal Health e-newsletter and flexible maintenance programs like her "15-minute fitness checkups".

With her outgoing nature and ability to create innovative programs to meet ever changing trends and client health fitness needs, Linda is well positioned to cast a fresh perspective on wellness programs, making and keeping them fun and continuously rewarding. She is a passionate master coach, supportive exercise trainer, presenter and business consultant, working with professionals, corporations and organizations to guide them in how to incorporate fitness into life.

To contact Linda, visit her website www.FitTraining.net or call (203) 877-5270.